17 Day Cookbook:

Delicious Healthy Weight Loss, Fat Loss and Flat Belly Recipes

By

Brittany Samons

Table of Contents

Introduction 6

1. Carrot and Apple Soup 8

2. Pomegranate Refresher 10

3. Apple Oat berry Smoothie 11

4. Chia Pudding 12

5. Crab Cakes with Citrus Vinaigrette 13

6. Preparing The Citrus Vinaigrette 14

7. Great Greens 15

8. Shrimp Cocktail 17

9. Roasted Vegetable Pizza 18

10. Low Fat Mini Cheesecakes 20

11. Over baked Chicken Fajitas 21

12. Grown Up Tuna Salad with Creamy Balsamic Dressing 22

13. Cool Chicken Lettuce Wraps 23

14. Mexican Chicken Dry Rub 25

15. Fruit Salsa 26

16. Grape and Lime Green Smoothie 27

17. Breakfast Smoothie 28

18. Broiled Tilapia with Parmesan 29

19. Chilled Mustard Potato 30

20. Spiced Thai Salad (Cucumber) 31

21. Spicy Corn & Black Bean Salad 32

22. Apple Coleslaw 33

23. Lunch Smoothie 34

24. Mock Mashed Potatoes..................................35

25. Roasted Sweet Potatoes...............................36

26. Sautéed Green Beans and Crimini Mushrooms 37

27. Salad in Jar (Mushrooms, Quinoa, Tomatoes, & Spinach) 39

28. Quinoa Salad with Black Beans, Cumin-Lime Dressing and Avocado 41

29. Parmesan Roasted Cauliflower.......................43

30. Strawberry Salad & Cool Cucumber 44

31. Strawberry Vinaigrette 45

32. Roasted Radishes with Baby Carrots 46

33. Broccoli Stir Fry and Tofu..............................47

34. Home-prepared Chili Con Carne Beans 48

35. Beef & Broccoli Stir Fry.................................49

36. French Onion Soup 50

Conclusion 51

Thank You Page 52

4

17 Day Diet Cookbook: Delicious Healthy Weight Loss, Fat Loss and Flat Belly Recipes

By Brittany Samons

Introduction

The 17 Day Diet is a diet plan that encourages the consumption of healthy foods while incorporating exercise and limiting starch and sugar. Divided into 4 different cycles, this diet will help you boost your metabolism, burn fat and create healthy new habits to lose excess weight. You will eat foods in unique cycles that last for seventeen days each to kick start your weight loss, and work toward a goal of maintaining a desired weight and eating healthfully for the rest of your life.

The 17 DD plan utilizes calorie cycling—varying your daily calorie intake—which has been shown to help the body in utilizing calories more efficiently by making sure that the metabolic rate does not have a chance to level out. It starts off as a mishmash of low fat and low carb, but mainly focuses on restricted calories. Nutritional experts the world over agree that restricting calories is crucial for weight loss.

There are recipes in the 17 Day Diet plan that can help you lose weight. This book advances a rundown of some of these delicious recipes. Read on for more.

1. Carrot and Apple Soup

Ingredients:

4 peeled carrots cut into quarter-inch pieces

Four cups non-fat vegetable broth, salt free/low
sodium

Salt and pepper to taste

Chopped chives or parsley, as garnish (if desired)

1 tsp. cumin or any other preferred spice

2 Tbsp. Olive Oil

1 chopped onion

1 Tbsp. garlic, chopped

2 peeled, diced and cored apples

Directions: Begin by heating olive oil in a medium sized
saucepan. Then, add onion, garlic and sauté till soft,
about four minutes. Then add carrots and apple and
sauté for two more minutes.

Add the cumin and vegetable broth and bring to a boil.
Minimize heat to simmer and cook till apples and
carrots all soften, about 15-20 minutes. Then remove

from heat and puree in batches in a blender.

Afterwards, season soup with pepper and salt...

Garnish with parsley or chives and serve.

2. Pomegranate Refresher

Ingredients:

1 cup ice

1 cup unsweetened pomegranate juice

1 cup unsweetened cranberry juice or strawberries

2 thinly sliced limes

1 bunch of fresh mint

Pomegranate seeds (if desired)

Ripe Kumquats, peeled

Instructions: Place ice in a punch bowl and add kumquats, cranberry juice, and pomegranate juice and stir properly. Then garnish with mint sprigs, lime slices and pomegranate seeds if desired. Serve.

Note: If using strawberries, blend kumquats and strawberries before adding pomegranate juice.

3. Apple Oat berry Smoothie

Ingredients:

Half cup of apple juice

A cup of strawberries

1 banana, peeled and chopped into chunks

1 peeled apple, cored and chopped into chunks

¼ cup quick cooking oats

Instructions: To core apples, chop whole apples into quarters. Chop away core and seeds from each quarter using a paring knife, beginning at the stem end and cutting downwards in a semi-circular motion. Place the cored apple and all other ingredients in a blender and blend until smooth and creamy. Garnish each serving with a drizzle of ground cinnamon.

4. Chia Pudding

Ingredients:

1 cup low-fat acidophilus milk or 1 cup Unsweetened Almond Milk, or soy milk

4 Tbsp. Chia Seeds

½ Tbsp. Cocoa powder

Pinch of Cinnamon

1/4 tsp. of real Vanilla

Dash Salt (optional)

Directions: Combine all the above ingredients in a small-mason jar with an air-tight lid and mix shake till ingredients are thoroughly mixed. Let it sit until Chia Seeds have absorbed majority of milk and have formed a pudding-like consistency. Monitor the pudding occasionally to shake up the mixture to ensure the cocoa is wholly incorporated. Be sure to top with your favorite fruit.

5. Crab Cakes with Citrus Vinaigrette

Ingredients:

Two 6 oz. cans of well drained Crab Meat

2 to 3 Tbsp. Olive oil

Wedges from half Lemon

One whisked egg white

Two Tbsp. Parmesan Cheese, Grated

Pepper to taste

Instructions: With this recipe, the key lies in ensuring the crab meat is perfectly drained. Thus, drain it very well before lightly flaking it in large mixing bowl. Then, whisk together 1 egg white and add to crab meat together with parmesan cheese. Proceed to blend together till it is perfectly combined.

Prepare four small patties. Heat 2 to 3 Tbsp. Olive Oil on in frying pan on medium heat. Then, brown each side for about ten minutes. Turn them carefully to avoid breaking.

Serve with Coleslaw and with Citrus Vinaigrette. Garnish with lemon wedges.

6. Preparing The Citrus Vinaigrette

Ingredients:

2 Tbsp. Olive Oil

Sweetener for taste

2 Tbsp. Freshly Squeezed orange juice

2 Tbsp. Apple Cider Vinegar

1 tsp. Dijon Mustard

Salt & Pepper to taste

Half bag of Coleslaw Mixture

Instructions: Whisk together all the above ingredients till well blended. Proceed to toss into coleslaw & serve with crab cakes. Use about 1 ½ bag of coleslaw mixture or more, depending on your desire. Serve for 2.

7. Great Greens

Ingredients:

1 bunch Swiss chard with leaves chopped, tough stems removed

1 large bunch kale, leaves dropped, tough stems & center ribs removed

1 tsp. dried basil

1 tsp. dill, dried

1 minced clove garlic

1 Tbsp. Fuhrman's Spicy Pecan Vinegar/any other flavored vinegar

1/2 Tbsp. Fuhrman's VegiZest/other salt-free seasoning blend, adjusted to taste

Black pepper to taste

Instructions: Begin by steaming the Swiss chard and kale together for seven minutes before transferring the steamed mixture to a separate bowl. Then, mix the remaining ingredients. Add this mixture to the greens. Add 2 to 3 Tbsp. of the steaming water for consistency, if desired. Serve for four.

8. Shrimp Cocktail

Ingredients:

Twelve oz. bag frozen and deveined small shrimp with tails removed

½ juiced Lemon

V8 tomato Juice

1 diced Avocado

2 deseeded and chopped Roma Tomatoes

1/2 lemon, chopped for garnish

1 Tbsp. diced red onion

2 Tbsp. chopped cilantro

Instructions: Begin by cleaning the shrimp and thawing it. Once thawed, combine tomatoes, avocado, shrimp, red onion cilantro, and juice of half of a lemon in a bowl. Then add V8 tomato- juice on mixture till it is completely covered. Let it chill for 1 to 2 hours. Use lemon wedge to garnish and serve for 4.

9. Roasted Vegetable Pizza

Ingredients:

2 cups broccoli florets

1 large sliced red bell pepper

1 tsp. garlic powder

1 Tbsp. balsamic vinegar

5 ounces baby spinach

1 large Portobello mushroom, chopped into half inch slices

Nutritarian Parmesan or 1 to 2 ounces non-dairy mozzarella

Half cup salt free or low sodium pasta sauce

Two (100 percent whole grain) tortillas or pita bread

1 tsp. Mrs. Dash seasoning or Salt free Spike seasoning

Directions: Begin by preheating your oven to 350 degrees Fahrenheit before tossing the bell pepper, broccoli, and mushrooms with balsamic vinegar, garlic powder, and seasoning. Then, roast seasoned veggies for about half an hour or until tender, occasionally turning and mounding to prevent them from drying. The spinach should be steamed till it wilts.

Bake the whole grain tortilla or pita bread directly on oven rack until it becomes crisp, seven minutes tops. Top your pita bread or tortilla with a thin layer of pasta sauce, and distribute roasted vegetables & spinach. Then, sprinkle with non-dairy mozzarella or Nutritarian Parmesan. Bake for another 3 to 5 minutes or till toppings are warm and cheese is melted, being careful enough so as not to brown the vegetables.

Note: Nutritarian Parmesan can be made by placing ¼ cup walnuts and ¼ cup nutritional yeast in a powerful processor and pulsing until the texture of grated Parmesan is realized. Be sure to store leftover in an air-tight container and place it in a refrigerator.

10. Low Fat Mini Cheesecakes

Ingredients:

One egg &1 beaten egg yolk

2 tsp. sweetener (Stevia)

Six oz. low-fat cream cheese (room temperature)

Half cup part skim ricotta cheese (room temperature)

1 tsp. vanilla extract

Directions: Preheat your oven to 350 degrees Fahrenheit. Spray regular size muffin pan with non-sticking spray. Place all in a large mixing bowl. Then beat with an electric mixer till mixture is smooth.

Divide batter evenly into six muffin cups then bake for about 30 minutes. Allow it to cool on the rack before gently removing mini cheesecakes from the pan. Top with your favorite berries. Serve for two.

11. Over baked Chicken Fajitas

Ingredients:

1/2 tsp. garlic powder

1/2 tsp. dried oregano

1/4 tsp. seasoned salt

1 lb. skinless, boneless chicken breasts, chopped into strips

2 Tbsp. Vegetable Oil like Extra Virgin Olive Oil

1 (15 oz.) can diced tomatoes with green chilies—Rotel

1 sliced medium sized onion

2 tsp. chili powder

1 1/2 tsp. cumin

1/2 red bell pepper, sliced into strips

half green bell pepper, sliced into strips

Directions: Preheat your oven to 400 degrees F. Next place chicken strips in a greased 13 by 9 inch baking dish. Then combine oil, cumin, chili powder, salt, dried oregano, and garlic powder in a small bowl. Drizzle the spice mixture over chicken & stir to coat. Then add the pepper, tomatoes, and onions to the dish & stir to combine. Then bake uncovered for 20 to 25 minutes or till chicken is cooked through & vegetables are tender.

12. Grown Up Tuna Salad with Creamy Balsamic Dressing

Creamy Balsamic Dressing

Ingredients:

1/4 cup balsamic vinegar

Dash of sweetener for taste

1/4 cup fat-free Greek yogurt

Directions: Whisk together all the ingredients. Refrigerate right away.

Grown up Tuna Salad

Ingredients:

Chopped Lettuce

1 to 2 Small quartered Tomatoes

1/8 cup fat-free crumbled feta cheese

1 small drained can tuna

Directions: Combine ingredients and toss in creamy balsamic dressing.

13. Cool Chicken Lettuce Wraps

Ingredients:

3.5 oz. minced chicken breast

half inch minced fresh ginger/dry, ground ginger

Minced green onion

Minced fresh garlic

1 Tbsp. Olive Oil

Directions: Over medium heat, add garlic, half of Olive Oil, onion and ginger and cook till soft. Then add remaining Olive Oil & minced chicken breast to pan & cook thoroughly.

To meat mixture, add the following:

1 tsp. of Asian red chili sauce or your preferred Chili Sauce

1 Tbsp. of wheat free Tamari sauce

1 Tbsp. rice wine vinegar

1 tsp. of Chinese five spice

Then cook for 5 minutes, stirring on low heat so as to largely reduce liquid. Next remove it from heat, and

23

spoon to whole lettuce leaves & roll—Boston lettuce, Bibb lettuce, and/or Iceberg are all great choices. Tamari can substitute Bragg Liquid Amino, but it introduces an entire different flavor to your dish. Be sure to top with bean sprouts for extra crunch.

14. Mexican Chicken Dry Rub

Ingredients:

1 tsp. cumin

1 tsp. oregano

1 tsp. garlic powder

1 tsp. chili powder

Olive Oil

Salt and pepper to taste

Prepare two chicken breasts as below:

Heat oil in pan over medium high heat... Sprinkle dry rub mixture generously on either side of chicken breasts. Then pan fry chicken until golden brown on one side on medium high; turn over, minimize heat to medium low, cover and cook till done. Slice chicken into thin strips.

15. Fruit Salsa

Ingredients:

1 Avocado, optional

Juice of half to one lemon for taste

One Sunburst Tomato

Zest of one lemon

2 to 3 Tbsp. of oil for taste

1 Roma Tomato

Half tsp. of Xylitol for taste

Salt and Pepper for taste

Directions: Cut up fruit in bite-size pieces. Add other ingredients and mix together thoroughly.
Next serve hot chicken over bed of lettuce & top with salsa.

16. Grape and Lime Green Smoothie

Ingredients:

1 cup fresh kale

Half peeled lime

1 ½ cup red-grapes

1 cup of water

Directions: Blend kale and water first. After it is well blended, add remaining ingredients and blend again.

17. Breakfast Smoothie

Ingredients:

One scoop vanilla whey protein powder

one serving powdered fiber

one cup unsweetened almond milk

½ cup plain low-fat yogurt

½ cup crush pineapple, canned in own juice, drained

½ frozen banana

Directions: Put the ingredients in a blender & blend till smooth. Blend the ingredients for several minutes to add air to the smoothie to make you feel fuller.

18. Broiled Tilapia with Parmesan

Ingredients:

4 Tilapia fillets, defrost if frozen

Quarter cup Parmesan Cheese

1/8 cup plain non-Fat/ low-fat Greek yogurt

1 Tbsp. Fresh Lemon Juice

Half tsp. fresh Dill

Pepper to taste

Directions: Turn broiler onto high & adjust oven rack to the top. Combine all ingredients except the tilapia in a small bowl. Set aside. Then place tilapia fillets on a foil-lined pan.

Broil for three minutes. Next remove from oven, flip over & apportion the Parmesan mixture over the uncooked sides of the tilapia. Then return to the oven and broil for an additional three to four minutes ensuring that the fish doesn't overcook. Serve for four.

19. Chilled Mustard Potato

Ingredients:

Three cubed Yukon Gold potatoes

3 cubed red potatoes

1/4 cup olive oil

3 Tbsp. apple cider vinegar

1 Tbsp. Dijon mustard

1/2 tsp. celery salt

1/4 tsp. pepper

Olive Oil for baking

Salt to taste

Directions: Preheat your oven to 375 degrees F. Mix celery salt, pepper, apple cider vinegar olive oil, and Dijon mustard in a small bowl. Then, arrange potatoes in a single layer on an oven safe pan and drizzle a few Tbsps. Over potatoes and mix properly.

Next bake in an oven for about 35 to 45 minutes or till fork is tender. Be sure to turn the potatoes after every 10 minutes to make sure that all sides are toasty. Then, remove from oven, cool, toss potatoes with mixture and serve accordingly.

20. Spiced Thai Salad (Cucumber)

Ingredients:

One Tbsp. Bragg liquid Aminos

One whole peeled cucumber, chopped julienne style

1/8 tsp. red chili flakes

Pepper and salt to taste

Stevia to taste

1 Tbsp. lemon juice...

1 Tbsp. green onion, chopped

a clove of garlic minced and crushed

one basil leaf sliced and rolled

1 tsp. chopped cilantro leaves

2 Tbsp. Olive Oil

Directions: Combine liquid ingredients including olive oil with the onion, garlic, chili flakes and fresh herbs. Mix julienned cucumbers & coat thoroughly with spice mixture. Then let marinate for ten minutes. Serve for one.

21. Spicy Corn & Black Bean Salad

Ingredients:

14 ounces (1 can) of rinsed and drained black beans (or your preferred beans)

two cups fresh corn kernels

one small seeded and chopped red bell pepper

1/2 chopped red onion

1 ½ tsp. ground cumin

1 ½ tsp. oregano

two tsp. hot sauce

one juiced lime

Two Tbsp. olive oil

Pepper and salt to taste

Directions: Mix all above ingredients in a bowl & allow them to stand fifteen minutes for flavors to combine. Toss and serve for 4 to 6.

22. Apple Coleslaw

Ingredients:

½ thinly sliced head cabbage

1 thinly sliced apple (leave few slices for garnish)

1 grated carrot

3 Tbsp. apple cider vinegar

2 to 4 Tbsp. non-fat plain yogurt

Pepper & salt to taste

Stevia to taste

Directions: Whisk together sweetener, apple cider vinegar, and non-fat plain yogurt till desired consistency is achieved. Then toss cabbage and carrot into mixture and let it marinate for about thirty minutes. Then add and apples and serve for one.

23. Lunch Smoothie

Ingredients:

1 cup of plain low-fat yogurt

1/3 cup of unsweetened soy milk or almond milk

one serving of vanilla whey protein in powder form

1 cup frozen strawberries

Truvia for taste

Powdered fiber, one serving

Directions: Put all the above ingredients in powerful blender, & blend till smooth and creamy. Freeze and serve for one.

24. Mock Mashed Potatoes

Ingredients:

½ tspn. of sliced fresh/dry chives to garnish

One medium head cauliflower

one Tbsp. non-fat Greek yogurt

¼ cup Parmesan, grated

½ tsp. garlic roasted or minced

1/2 tsp. sea salt

1/8 tspn. of ground black pepper, fresh

Directions: Set stockpot of water to boil on high heat. Then clean and cut cauliflower into tiny pieces. Next cook in boiling water for approx. six minutes or till done. Then drain water, and immediately pat cooked cauliflower very dry between various layers of paper towel.

In a food processor, puree the hot cauliflower with non-fat Greek yogurt, garlic, pepper, Parmesan and salt till smooth. Next, garnish with chives. Make 2 to 3 servings.

25. Roasted Sweet Potatoes

Ingredients:

One medium size peeled sweet Potato, cut into half inch cubes

1 Tbsp. olive oil

Pepper and Salt to taste

Directions: Preheat your oven to 400 Degrees. Then put cut sweet-potatoes on baking sheet and drizzle with salt, pepper and olive oil. Next, toss to fully coat. Then bake for 35 to 40 minutes till done. Make 1 to 2 servings.

26. Sautéed Green Beans and Crimini Mushrooms

Ingredients:

1 lb. trimmed and chopped into half green beans

Salt &Pepper, to taste

two Tbsp. olive oil

½ chopped onion (If desired)

1 minced garlic clove

1/2 carton of crimini mushrooms, sliced

1/4 cup of salt free, and fat free vegetable broth

Instructions: Steam the fresh green beans over medium heat till about to fork tender. Then drain the steamed green beans, cover & put aside. Add onions, oil and minced garlic to pan over medium heat and sauté two to three minutes. Then add mushrooms and season with pepper and salt.

Next, sauté the mushrooms three to five minutes with onions before adding green beans back to pan. Then heat green beans through and add vegetable broth then cook for one to two minutes. Transfer green beans & mushrooms to your serving plate. Serve for 3 to 4.

27. Salad in Jar (Mushrooms, Quinoa, Tomatoes, & Spinach)

Ingredients:

1 cup quinoa, cooked

two big handfuls spinach

one cup mushrooms, chopped

one cup cherry tomatoes

1/2 diced red onion

4 Tbsp. low-fat balsamic Vinaigrette or homemade one utilizing Balsamic Vinegar, seasonings and Olive oil

Be sure to layer ½ of each ingredient in Mason jar like bellow:

Dressing

Onion

Tomatoes

Mushrooms

Quinoa

Spinach

Note: If you want to keep your salads in a jar fresh, ensure that the dressing is always on the bottom and salad greens topping it.

28. Quinoa Salad with Black Beans, Cumin-Lime Dressing and Avocado

Ingredients:

One cup of rinsed dry quinoa

1 Tbsp. olive oil

1 ¾ cup water

One can of drained and rinsed black beans

One avocado, chopped into chunks

handful of quartered cherry tomatoes

½ diced red onion

One small minced clove garlic

One red bell pepper, chopped into chunks

Small handful diced cilantro

Dressing:

1 juiced lime

½ Tbsp. cumin

½ Tbsp. olive oil

Salt to taste

Directions: Warm the olive oil in medium size saucepan on medium heat. Then add the rinsed quinoa & toast for about 2 to 3 minutes till it starts smelling nutty. Then add water, stir once, cover, and simmer with lid for twenty minutes. While quinoa is cooking, prepare all other ingredients.

Make the dressing by mixing oil, cumin, lime juice, and salt. Whisk aggressively before adjusting seasoning as desired. Upon quinoa finishing cooking, remove from heat and fluff with fork. Then add black beans & toss to warm them through. Allow quinoa to cool for approx. 5 minutes before adding all remaining ingredients—including the dressing—and mix. You may adjust seasoning if necessary.

29. Parmesan Roasted Cauliflower

Ingredients:

6 ounces (1 1/2) cups cauliflower florets

2 tsp. grated low-fat Parmesan cheese

1 tsp. fresh parsley leaves, chopped

1/4 tsp. garlic powder

¼ tsp. ground black pepper

Salt to taste

1 tsp. extra-virgin olive oil

Directions: Preheat your oven to 425 degrees. Combine the garlic powder, pepper, cheese, parsley and cauliflower in a medium size bowl. Season with salt and toss to mix. Season with salt and toss to mix.

Then drizzle on the oil and toss again before transferring the mixture to a small non-sticking baking dish. Next, bake for about 17 minutes, tossing until lightly browned and crisp tender. Make sure that you serve immediately.

30. Strawberry Salad & Cool Cucumber

Ingredients:

One serving of strawberry vinaigrette

Stevia for taste

5 to 6 cut strawberries

Chopped Mint (optional)

Ground white pepper, fresh

One whole sliced cucumber

Directions: Chop cucumber & strawberries. Then add dressing, pepper and stevia to taste. Next, let it marinate for 10 minutes at least.

31. Strawberry Vinaigrette

Ingredients:

5 to 5 medium sized strawberries

1 Tbsp. apple cider vinegar

1 Tbsp. lemon juice

1 Tbsp. Olive Oil

Dash of salt

Dash of cayenne (if desired)

Fresh ground black pepper to taste

Stevia to taste

Water for consistency

Instructions: Mix all ingredients in a powerful food processor and puree till smooth. Then pour over fresh green salad and garnish with sliced strawberries and freshly chopped black pepper.

32. Roasted Radishes with Baby Carrots

Ingredients:

1 bunch small-to-medium radishes, about 12

twelve baby carrots

1 Tbsp. olive oil

1 tsp. thyme, dried

Pepper and salt to taste

Half Lemon

Instructions: Preheat your oven to 450 Degrees Fahrenheit. Then place the carrots and radishes on a baking sheet and toss with thyme, olive oil, pepper and salt. Next, roast till tender yet firm in the center, approx. 25 minutes. Lastly, squeeze with a little lemon juice before serving for four.

33. Broccoli Stir Fry and Tofu

Ingredients:

One package extra firm tofu

3 to 4 small heads of cut and steamed broccoli

Two Tbsp. Bragg Liquid Aminos

Pepper, salt and Garlic Powder to taste

Red Chili Flakes to taste

1 Tbsp. Olive Oil

Instructions: In large skillet, heat olive oil. Then cut tofu into rectangular (half inch thick by half one and a half inch thick). Next, lay the tofu on paper towel so as to drain any excess water present. Then season the water free tofu with pepper, salt & garlic powder. Afterwards, fry seasoned tofu in sizeable pan till golden brown & crisp outside. Then add steamed broccoli to tofu in pan and add red chili flakes and liquid Aminos... Serve when hot for three.

34. Home-prepared Chili Con Carne Beans

Ingredients:

1 lb. 7pc fat ground Sirloin

2 chopped tomatoes

One tsp. cumin

One tsp. chili powder to taste

One tsp. oregano

Garlic & onion powder to taste

1/4 cup of beef broth, organic

1 tsp. agave sweetener

One can of El Pato spiced tomato sauce

one can of rinsed Pinto/black beans, use water to rinse

Salt & pepper for taste

Instructions: Brown the sirloin, add chopped tomatoes & spices & simmer for a couple of minutes. Then put El Pato tomato sauce, beans, beef broth, beef and agave sweetener. Simmer for about twenty minutes. Serve for four.

35. Beef & Broccoli Stir Fry

Ingredients:

One small Sirloin steak, cooked and chopped into thin slices

Half cup of cooked brown rice

1 whole beaten egg

1 tsp. oil

1 Tbsp. Bragg Liquid Aminos/light soy sauce

Salt and pepper to taste

One cup of steamed broccoli florets

Quarter cup of frozen peas—slightly thawed (if desired)

Red Chili Flakes to taste

Instructions: Over high heat, heat skillet, add oil and reduce to medium high. Then, add meat and rice, and cook till warmed through. Next, add beaten egg to pan and cook till egg is properly done. Then add peas and broccoli and warm through. Next add Bragg Liquid, pepper, salt and red chili flakes. Serve for 1 while hot.

36. French Onion Soup

Ingredients:

Whole thinly sliced onion

1/4 lb. thinly sliced beef

Non-fat, low-sodium beef/vegetable broth

1 roasted and minced garlic clove

Pepper and salt

3 Tbsp. low-fat Mozzarella Cheese

Instructions: Put the onions into an oven-proof saucepan and add enough broth that it covers half the onions. Then cook till onions are tender. Next, season with pepper and salt to taste.

Preheat the broiler, then add thinly chopped beef to the onions and broil for about five minutes. Then top with mashed roasted garlic & mozzarella cheese and broil again for 5 minutes till cheese begins to brown. Serve for one.

Conclusion

The 17 Day Diet offers direction for a wholesome way of eating that's sustainable—it is clean, incorporates lean proteins, healthy carbs, healthy fats, and eradicates fried and processed foods. When you follow aforementioned recipes and incorporate exercise, you will lose weight in a healthy way without having to starve. What is more, it can be adapted to a wide range of cuisines, from Chinese to Tex Mex & everything in between.

Thank You Page

I want to personally thank you for reading my book. I hope you found information in this book useful and I would be very grateful if you could leave your honest review about this book. I certainly want to thank you in advance for doing this.

If you have the time, you can check my other books too.

CPSIA information can be obtained
at www.ICGtesting.com
Printed in the USA
BVHW041125030121
596871BV00025B/2492